Back Pain Solution

*Live Life Again With This Proven Back
Pain Cure Without Drugs Or Surgery*

CRISTINA ABATE

Disclaimer

CONTENTS

INTRODUCTION

I want to thank you and congratulate you for buying this book, *"Back Pain Solution"*.

This book contains proven steps and strategies on how to live life again without drugs or surgery.

For example, in this book you will learn what exactly back pain is, how many types of back pain are there, as well as the different causes of back pain.

You will also learn how to avoid back pain, how to sit correctly to minimize the stress on your back, and also different exercises that will help you avoid and prevent back pain.

You will also learn different ways in which you can relieve back pain, like using dry heat and moist heat, and much more.

Thanks again for purchasing this book, I hope you enjoy it!

CHAPTER 1

WHAT IS BACK PAIN?

Back pain is one of the most common health problems around the world. In the United States, 8 out of 10 people are affected by it at one point or another in their lives.

One of the main reasons of back pain is the ageing process, which is why it is more common in people who are between 40 to 80 years of age; it is also more common in women than in men.

As we age and grow older, our bodies become weaker and the odds of experiencing pain in the lower back due to spinal degeneration or disc diseases increase.

Although it is not always known what the cause of back pain is, lifestyle is often one of the most important factors in causing it.

For instance, people who have sedentary lifestyles or jobs that require them to sit on a chair and work on a computer for long periods of time are especially susceptible to back pains.

A survey revealed that 1/4th of all the people over the age of 18 in the United States said that they have had back pain within the last 90 days that lasted for at least 24 hours or more; 7.6% of them also said that they have had at least one episode of severe acute low-back pain within the last year.

According to another survey conducted by National Institute of Health Statistics, pain in the lower back is the most common problem people face, followed by headaches/migraines and neck pains.

It has been reported that the adults who suffer from lower back pain are usually in worse mental and physical conditions than those who do not suffer from it. 28% of the people with lower back pain reported that their activities were limited because of their condition being chronic.

Having lower back pain also increases the chances of other problems, and it was found that people with lower back pain were thrice as likely to be in a poor health condition and also 4 times as likely to go through severe mental distress as someone without low back pain.

Smokers were also found likely to have back pain.

Another study revealed that sleep disturbance is common in more than half the people having back pain.

Back pain, as the name suggests, is the pain in the back.

There are three main types of back pains, which are:

- Upper back pain
- Middle back pain
- Lower back pain

Symptoms:

Following are the common symptoms experienced by people who have back pain:

- Muscle spasms and pain in the back when standing, often making it difficult to stand.
- Pain in the back going all the way from the lower back to hips, the back of thighs, and to the calves and toes.
- A recurring lower back or middle back pain, especially after prolonged periods of inactivity or standing or sitting for long times.
- Severe pain localized in the lower, middle, or upper back, or in the neck, especially after lifting heavy weights or performing other laborious actions and activities.

- Pain, stiffness, or ache in any part of your spine, all the way from the tail bone to the base of your neck.

Note: Sometimes pain in the upper back is also a symptom of having a heart attack.

CHAPTER 2

CAUSES OF BACK PAIN

Usually the back pain is either caused by ageing or a person's lifestyle.

Severe to short-term back pain lasts anywhere from a few days to a few weeks.

Other than that, back pain is caused by injuries, accidents, arthritis, or traumas.

Sometimes it is also caused by a sudden strenuous activity or jolts, or anything else that stresses the spine.

The symptoms of back pain range from an inability to stand or sit to rigidity, limited flexibility, and pangs of back in the back.

Back pain can also be the result of pain being radiated from another part of the body.

The chronic back pains are progressive and need to be treated, or else they can get worse.

Following are the common causes of back pains:

Muscle Strains

A muscle strain, also called a pulled muscle, is when the muscles of the back are over-stretched or torn. This is usually caused by heavy lifting or exercising so hard that the muscle fibres get damaged.

Lumbar Sprain
A lumbar sprain is when the ligaments (the tough and flexible tissues connecting bones, cartilages, or holding joints together) are over-stretched or torn. The over-stretched or torn ligaments cause the tissues to become inflamed which results in pain in the back.

Sciatica Pain
Pain in the back is also caused when something presses on the sciatic nerve, like a bulging or ruptured disk.

Usually it only affects on side, and the pain goes down the lower back to one leg; sometimes it can go down to the foot or toes as well, but that depends on where the sciatic nerve is being pressed.

Sometimes the sciatic pains are minor and infrequent, and at others they are constant and acute.

Work
Your work can also be a cause of your back pain: people who have jobs that require sitting on a chair and working on desks all day, heavy lifting, or strenuous activity that can twist the spine.

Sitting on chairs that are not comfortable or slouchy postures also lead to back pain.

Bags
Bags are often responsible for back pain. Heavy bags, briefcases, or even large purses with loads of heavy items in them can cause stress on the back and lead to pulled or over-stretched muscles.

Herniated Disc
There are gel like discs in your spine that keep it cushioned. As you age, or due to injuries, these discs can become weak or bulge, and such discs can put additional pressure on the nerve roots in your spine and cause pain.

Chronic Conditions
Back pain is also caused by several chronic conditions like Spinal Stenosis, Spondylitis, Fibromyalgia, etc.

Being Overweight

People who are overweight are very likely to experience back pain. The additional weight in the body, particular in the middle, puts extra stress on the back by shifting your centre of gravity. Ideally you should try to keep your weight 10 pounds below the recommended weight to stave off back problems.

Smoking

Cigarettes contain nicotine, an alkaloid that restricts the flow of blood in your body. We already know that smoking causes impotence, chiefly by restricting blood flow, but it also restricts the flow of blood to the discs in your back. It prevents the new bone growth and negatively affects the absorption of calcium in the body, thereby increasing the chances of getting back pain and injuries.

Sedentary Lifestyle

When people limit their movements, whether due to job or some pain, they are at an increased risk of pain. This is because your blood flow increases when you are active, but having a sedentary lifestyle means that the flow of blood to the affected area will be limited, thereby putting you at an increased risk of experiencing pain.

Posture

Your posture plays a vital role in how much stress is placed on your back, and can even change the anatomical characteristics of your spine. For instance, when you are sitting on a chair with your legs dangling down, you are putting extra stress on your back. Incorrect postures increase the chances of back pain and injuries.

Lifting Weights Incorrectly

While working out is good, and you may have to lift weights while you do so, lifting weights incorrectly can actually have severe consequences. When you suddenly lift a heavy weight, or try to lift more weight than you actually can, your back has to pay the price by supporting it all and going under extreme stress; this is when the muscles mostly get over-stretched or torn.

Lack of Exercise

According to Nancy E. Epstein, MD, chief of neurosurgical spine, "The failure to perform any exercise, particularly abdominal strengthening exercises, may lead to poor posture and increased low back pain." Exercises for back pain include those that can strengthen your core, like Pilates.

CHAPTER 3

HOW TO RELIEVE BACK PAIN

Back pain, whether acute or minor, can mess up your day.

The additional stress on the back can exhaust and tire you within minutes and hinder your progress in whatever you are doing.

Since the back pain has a high potential of getting worse and becoming chronic, it is important to pay attention to it and relieve it.

How and when you treat your back pain determines how long it will last and how quickly you will recover from it and get better.

There are many ways in which you can relieve pain, but the best methods are those that can cure it without you having to use any medicines or pills.

Following are some of the healthy ways in which back pain can be cured, treated, and relieved:

Exercise
The back and abdominal muscles play a vital role in supporting your spine. Usually these muscles do not get enough exercise daily so they become unhealthy.

More than half the people who experience back pain wish that they had exercised more in the past to prevent the pain.

The exercises for back pain include exercises like Pilates or others that work on the core muscles. You can easily train your back muscles and strengthen your back by exercising for 20 minutes daily. Following are some exercises for your back:

The Pelvic Tilt
To perform this exercise you should lie on the floor and bend your knees. Put your arms on your sides and keep your feet parallel to each other. Then, without using the muscles of your legs or hips, tighten the abs muscles by pulling your lower back and navel towards the floor, and then hold the position for five seconds. Repeat this exercise ten times.

The Trunk Curl
To perform this exercise you should lie on the floor and bend your knees, and cross your arms on your chest. Then engage the upper abs by slightly lifting your upper body off the floor, about 15 degrees. Hold this position for five seconds before lowering your upper body to the floor again. Repeat this exercise ten times.

Leg Lifts
To perform this exercise you need to stand in a swimming pool. Stand close to the side wall of the pool and place a hand on its edge, then raise one leg straight and slowly to the front, and then lower it slowly. Repeat this exercise ten times, 5 times for each leg.

These are only a few exercises and you can try many more that can strengthen the core muscles. Some of them will be mentioned later.

Heat Therapy
One of the causes of back pain is the inadequate blood flow, and that pain can be relieved by increasing the blood flow. You can increase the blood flow with heat therapy because it also inhibits the pain messages that your back sends to your brain.

It is especially helpful in relieving lower back pain. Heat therapy is very easy and can be performed in many different ways, with dry heat as well as moist heat.

When performing heat therapy with dry heat, you can use heating pads, saunas, electronic heating pads, etc., while heat therapy with moist heat includes steamed towels, heating packs, as well as taking hot baths. Ideally, you should experiment with both dry heat and moist heat to see which one works best for you.

Gel Packs

Most gel packs can be used hot or cold. You can microwave a gel pack, or put it in hot water, to heat it up and then apply it to your lower back for immediate relief.

Hot/Steam Baths

Hot/steam baths and saunas promote relaxation and ease your body, as well as improve the blood flow to the affected areas.

Heat Wrap

A heat wrap has the added benefit that it can easily be wrapped around the waist and can continuously provide heat for a long period of time. You can also use hot water bottles, as they can stay hot or warm for about half an hour.

Sleep

Restorative sleep can also help in reliving back pain. The only problem with this is that more than half of the people who have back pain also suffer from sleep disturbance, which makes it hard for them to get restorative sleep. To prevent this, try relaxation and other techniques that can aid you in sleeping.

Back Massage

A back massage is also an excellent way of relieving back pain and promoting blood circulation in the back. You can ask your masseuse to knead the muscles in your back to get maximum benefit from the massage.

Mattress

Your mattress is often the cause of back pain, especially if it is old and saggy, so get a new mattress instead. There are new mattresses available that are especially designed for the back.

Yoga

Yoga is also a healthy exercise. It helps you relax while giving you a workout at the same time. It engages most of the muscles in your body so the blood flow is promoted while your body relaxes.

CHAPTER 4

EAT HEALTHY TO AVOID BACK PAIN

Some studies link back pain to our diets, which means that we can beat back pain by eating healthy foods. Avoid eating foods that are rich in saturated fats or contain vegetable oils.

There are certain foods that you should avoid, and others that you should eat less to avoid back pain. And then there are foods that you 'should' eat to promote the health of your back.

Foods to Avoid
Avoid all the processed foods, if possible. This includes most microwavable meals, hot dogs, and bars of snacks that contain corn syrup with high fructose or sugar.

Also avoid all sodas whether they are diet or not. Wheat, eggs, and dairy can also cause back pain.

Foods to Eat Less
If you can't completely avoid the foods, you should eat them less often. There are some foods that you shouldn't eat too often, and, if you do, you should reduce your intake. These foods include:

- Fast food bars that contain a high amount of sugar
- Artificial sugars

- Pops and diet pops
- Foods that contain a high amount of saturated fats
- Margarine
- Trans fats
- Vegetable shortening
- Processed foods
- High-fructose corn syrup

Foods that You Should Eat

Pain naturally causes us to become stiff so our muscles become tight, which may increase the pain, but it can be avoided by eating foods that can actually help our muscles relax. Foods that contain a high amount of magnesium, like spinach, salmon, bananas, or eggplants can help relax the muscles and reduce pain.

You should try to include these foods in your diet, especially if you have back pain; these foods include:

- Fish, like salmon, albacore white tuna and canned sardines
- Ginger, turmeric, garlic, onions and black pepper
- Leafy vegetables such as broccoli, cauliflower, cabbage and brussels sprouts
- Fruits and berries like pomegranate, banana, organic cherries, etc.
- Rosemary, basil and fennel
- Olive oil
- Nuts, including pecans and almonds
- Green tea

CHAPTER 5

EXERCISES FOR BACK PAIN

You can relive back pain, or avoid it altogether, by excising regularly for at least 20 minutes per day.

Most of the people who experience back pain said that they wish they had exercised in the past, and would have definitely done it if they knew how painful back pain was going to be.

So, whether you have back pain or not, it is recommended that you start excising regularly to avoid back pain in the future.

Below are some videos of exercises which will help alleviate the pain:

https://www.youtube.com/watch?v=dATOtllZA2I

https://www.youtube.com/watch?v=FVtNLwundu4

https://www.youtube.com/watch?v=2Pmknfjq89U

https://www.youtube.com/watch?v=SuScgzVJp-s

https://www.youtube.com/watch?v=CO3racIlTcg

Following are some easy to perform exercises for back pain:

Seated Thoracic Rotations

This exercise is for the upper spine. It gives you more control over your spine while increasing its flexibility and making it mobile. This exercise can be done in as little as 5 minutes.

You can start this exercise by sitting on a stable and solid surface like a chair without a backrest. Your feet should touch the floor so you can have a better grip. Close your legs so that your knees are touching. Sit alert and tall as you would sit on a chair with a back. Next, put both of your hands behind your head. You may interlock your fingers but you must not lean your head on your hands for support.

Stretch your elbows back and straighten your chest. Rotate all the way to your left side through your chest, but your lower belly should not move as the rotation is going to be in the upper part of your back. When you have reached as far as you easily can, hold the position for a second or two. Before you return to your starting position, bend to the side while your chest is pulled up. Rotate back to the main position, and then repeat the same steps for the right side. Perform at least 8 repetitions for each side while alternating between the sides.

Note: When performing a spinal exercise, never push yourself too hard. Injuries to the spine may result in complete loss of sensory and motor functions, so do not push yourself too hard to avoid injury. Flexibility and mobility increase with regular exercise.

Supine Spinal Twists

This exercise works on your shoulder muscles and spine, and can be performed in less than 15 minutes.

You can start this exercise by lying down on your back. Then bend your legs by raising your feet to 90-degree angles so that your calves are parallel to the ground. With your legs bent, stretch your arms with palms facing downwards. This will be your core position for this exercise. Then slowly, with your knees joined together, lower your legs to the right side of your body but make sure they do not touch the ground. Stay in this position for about 30 seconds and then return to your core position.

Repeat the same exercise as above, but lower your legs to the left side of your body and alternate between both sides. Repeat five times for each side.

Hamstring Stretch

You can start this exercise by lying on your back and bending one knee.

Then straighten your knee (this can be done by looping a towel under your foot and then pulling on the towel). When you straighten your leg, you will actually feel your hamstring stretching. Hold this position for 15 seconds, and repeat thrice for each leg.

Press-up Back Extensions
You can begin this exercise by lying on your stomach and with your hands under your shoulders. Start by pushing with both hands to lift your shoulders off the floor. You can also put your elbows on the floor, underneath your shoulders, and hold this position for 5 seconds. Repeat 5-10 times.

Bottom to Heels Stretch
You can start this exercise by getting on all fours. Your hands should be under your shoulders and your knees should be under your buttocks. Do not lock your elbows or overarch your back; keep your neck straight and long. Then start by slowly moving your hips backwards while maintaining the natural curve position of the spine, and hold the position for 5 seconds before returning to the original position. Repeat five times.

Deep Abdominal Strengthening
You can start performing this exercise by lying on your back. Use a small cushion for your head. Then bend your knees while keeping them hip width apart. Tuck your chin in and relax, then begin exercise by exhaling. As you exhale, draw the muscles of your lower abs and pelvis upwards, and hold this position for ten seconds; breathe while you hold this position. Repeat this ten times.

Bird Dog
You can start performing this exercise by getting on all fours and tightening the muscles of your stomach. Then lift one leg behind you and extend it, and hold this position for five seconds; make sure that your leg stays in level with your hips. Then return to the starting position and repeat the same exercise for your other leg. As you continue the repetitions, try to hold each position for longer than before. To get the most benefit from this exercise, when you lift and extend a leg, also try to lift and raise its opposite arm. Maintain the position of your lower back, but do not sag or overarch it.

CHAPTER 6

CORRECTING YOUR POSTURE TO AVOID BACK PAIN

People who work in offices, have desk jobs or other jobs that require sitting for extended periods of time, tend to experience back ache more often than others and are at an increased risk of sustaining back injuries.

The aches in the lower back and spine can be acute, severe, and debilitating. The back pain can only be tolerated if it is minor and infrequent, but at a certain stage it starts limiting your activities. It makes you restless, lose concentration, and unable to focus on your work.

There is always a chance that back ache will become chronic and turn into something worse, especially among people working desk jobs or sitting at incorrect postures.

It would be wise to correct the posture of your back rather than spend a lot of money on medical bills afterwards. The spinal surgeries are complicated and one of the most expensive ones, and often with a low success rate.

When you sit in the same position for an extended time, your body puts an extra amount of stress on your spine, but you can easily avoid it by correcting the posture of your back and your sitting position.

You can work for a long time and avoid backache and stress by sitting correctly. Here's how to do it the right way:

Support the Upper and Lower Back

When selecting a chair for work, go for one that can support your entire back. When you are working long hours, press your back into the back rest to keep your back supported and release stress from it. Most desk chairs only have a support for the upper back, but whether or not you have a back problem, get one with support for the entire back. There is a slight arch in the back and it can't be supported with a straight chair, so unless your chair is specifically designed to support the arch in the back, use a cushion as it will support the lower back.

Adjusting your Work Area

The placement of your chair and table also plays a crucial role and affects your back. While chairs and desks come in standard heights, people do not, and therefore the requirements are different for everyone. You should adjust your table and chair in such a way that when you are sitting or working, the screen of your monitor or laptop should be right in front of you, a little below your eye level. The correct sitting position and adjustment will put your gaze in the middle of the screen, minimising the stress. Adjust your chair according to your height so that your feet are resting on the floor instead of dangling in the air.

The Placement of your Keyboard

Since you use your hands when using your keyboard, an additional weight is put on your back. You can minimise it by opting for a chair that comes with armrests, and placing your keyboard in such a way that you can easily type on it while your arms rest on the armrests. Keep the keyboard 4 to 6 inches away from yourself, at a comfortable distance.

Keep your Feet on the Floor

If your chair is too low, your knees will be above the base of your spine and put an additional weight on it, just like dangling feet can if your chair is too high. Both of these positions can put extra weight and stress on your lower back and the spine. It can be hard to actually feel this pressure because we are used to our own body weight and barely notice it, if we ever do. Sit in a correct posture by adjusting your seat so that your feet are resting comfortably on the floor.

Take 5-Minute Breaks

It is also very important to take breaks from sitting regularly. The blood flow decreases if you continue sitting in the same position, so take a walk or go for a short run after every hour or two of sitting. Breaks can be as short as 5 minutes and can provide the much needed exercise and change, and restore the blood flow in your body.

CHAPTER 7

RELAXING TO REDUCE BACK ACHE

One of the causes of back pain is tight muscles.

Our muscles tighten when we are in pain or stressed.

This can be avoided by relaxing our bodies. One of the easiest and most popular ways of relaxing is meditation, as it not only helps relax the body and the muscles but also reduces stress and promotes positive thinking. You can meditate for as little as 15 minutes per day.

Here's how to meditate:

The only thing you need for meditation is a quiet room.

When selecting a room or place for meditation, try to find a place that has the least disturbance and noise.

Since meditation requires focus and concentration, avoid places where someone can disturb you.

Silence is preferred for meditation but natural voices like those of birds, ocean, etc. are also helpful.

You can also play some meditative music to help you relax and concentrate, or just focus on emptying your mind.

There are some meditative mantras that you can chant to improve your focus. 'Om' is one of the most popular meditative mantras as it is deeply resonant and easy to pronounce when meditating.

You have to let the music fill your mind and give yourself to it. Relax and give your mind a break.

If you want, you can run the events of your day through your mind and see what you could have done differently to make things better.

You can also think about the things that lie ahead and that maybe bothering you.

When your mind is calm and tranquil, it is easier to find a better solution to your problems.

You can meditate for as long as you want, but it is recommended that you meditate for at least 15 minutes, four days a week.

When you finish meditating, do not try to get up quickly. Slowly transition and take in things, open your eyes and return your breathing to its normal pace, and get up slowly. Do not rush, for that is not what meditation is about.

When you concentrate on yourself or on something aside from your pain, your pain goes away.

Whether you are an optimist, pessimist, or a realist, when you think positive, you are happier and relaxed.

If you find the glass half-full, when you drink, it may not quench your thirst but it will surely leave you feeling more satisfied.

That can be applied to all scenarios of life, the way you look at them defines how they will affect you, so, start thinking positive and relax.

It may take some time but with practice and patience you can meditate to reduce your pain and relax your body.

CONCLUSION

Thank you again for purchasing this book!

I hope this book was able to help you free yourself from back pain.

I appreciate you for taking the time out of your day or evening to read this book, and if you have an extra second, I would love to hear what you think about this book by leaving a review on Amazon. I would greatly appreciate it!

Go to http://amzn.to/1t8J7ze

If the links do not work, for whatever reason, you can simply search for the title "Back Pain Solution" on the Amazon website.

Thank you again, and I wish you nothing but the best!

Cristina Abate

HERE IS A BOOK I RECOMMEND CALLED
"FOLLOW YOUR OWN PATH"

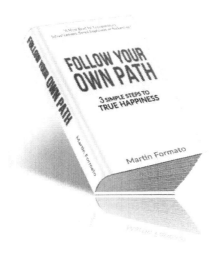

This is the coolest book I have ever read and by purchasing a copy you put another copy into the hands of someone less fortunate as the author's mission which is to inspire people to do what they love that also contributes to humanity. That is a win/win/win.

Who Is This Book For?

This book is for anyone who is hungry.

Anyone who wants more out of life.

Anyone who knows that they have more to give, share and experience.

Anyone who feels deep down, in their heart, that they are here for a reason.

It's a book for people who feel stuck, lost, depressed or even suicidal.

In particular, it's for, entrepreneurs who are struggling, school leavers who are lost, employees who are bored or in a job they hate and redundees who feel discarded.

Today, more than ever in history, people need more direction and less information.

This book will put you on the right path, YOUR PATH.

Who Is This Book NOT For?

You should not get this book until you are certain that you truly wish to change your life and you are 100 percent committed to it.

Ask yourself these 2 questions:

1. Do I want to make a change voluntarily, completely of my own choice?
2. Do I really want to change my life?

If you cannot honestly say "Yes" without hesitation to both questions, then it is better that you wait until you are serious about changing your life.

As one monk famously said "We want only warriors... victims need not apply".

Go to: http://amzn.to/2kQC9CK

If the links do not work, for whatever reason, you can simply search for the title "Follow Your Own Path" on the Amazon website.

CONTENTS FROM THE BOOK
"FOLLOW YOUR OWN PATH"

STEP 3: GIVE YOUR PASSION TO THE WORLD

Give Your Passion To The World

How Do I Start?

Planning To Live Passionately

10 Reasons Why You MUST Set Goals

Guidelines To Goal Setting

Setting Goals

Time Bound Goals

Prioritize Your Goals

Make Your Goals SMARTER

Your Life Plan On A Page

Milestones

Actions And Tasks

Goal Achievement Plan

Weekly Timetable

Things To Do Today

Living Passionately

14 Reasons Why People Don't Achieve Their Goals

Motivation And Focus

Conclusion

Resources

About The Author

Go to http://amzn.to/2kQC9CK

If the links do not work, for whatever reason, you can simply search for the title "Follow Your Own Path" on the Amazon website.

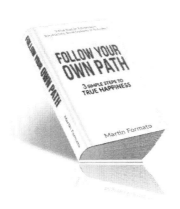

BONUS: FREE BOOK

Go to the website at www.DoingWorkThatMatters.com and enter your email address to get the FREE book "**Find Your Gift, Passion and Purpose**".

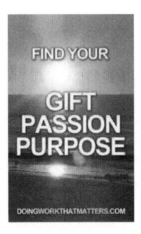

Once you register you will be sent FREE information that will further help you create a life you love.

All you have to do is enter your email address to get instant access.

This information will help you get more out of your life – to be able to reach your goals, have more motivation, be at your best, and live the life you have always dreamed of.

New resources are continually added, which you will be notified of as a subscriber. These will help you live your life to the fullest!

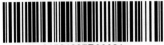

Printed in Great Britain
by Amazon